UNDERSTANDING ZIKA: A Guide For Researchers
Finding needles in the haystack
Seeing that which cannot be seen

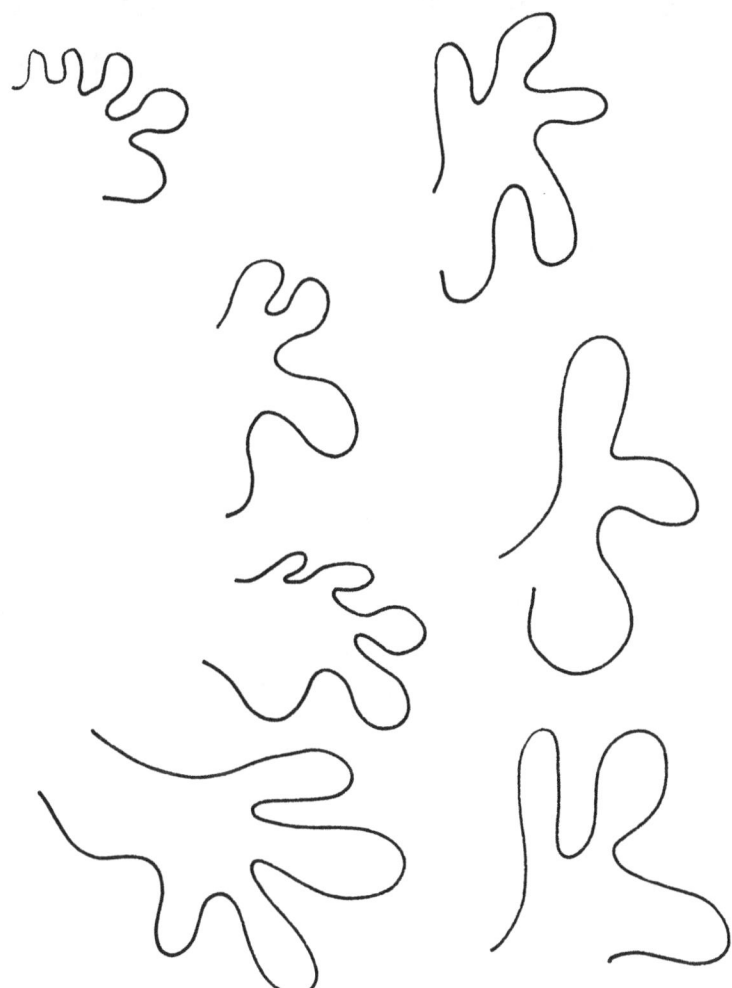

Camilia MacPherson, Ph.D., D.Th.
2016

INTRODUCTION

This book is written using Automatic Drawings and Surreal Art. All pages must be viewed from every angle and varying depths including 'thumb nails.' The diagram below indicates the pre-calligraphy graphics used in this book. There is no top or bottom of the page.

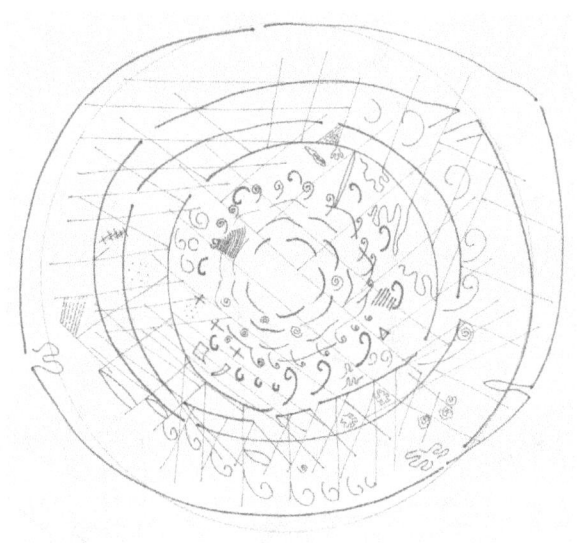

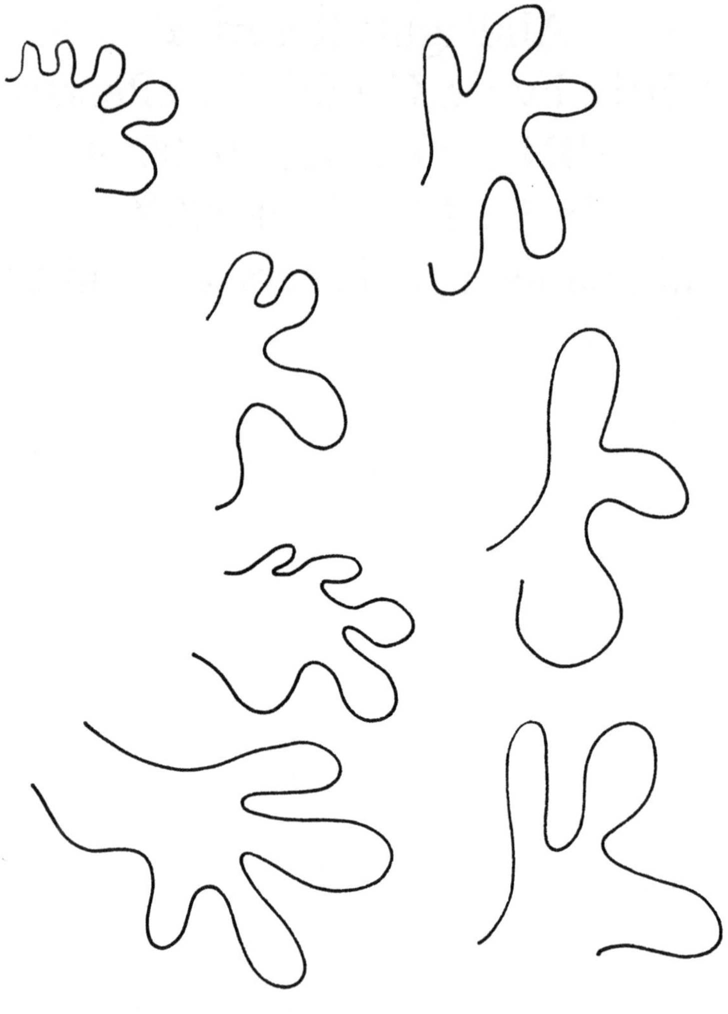

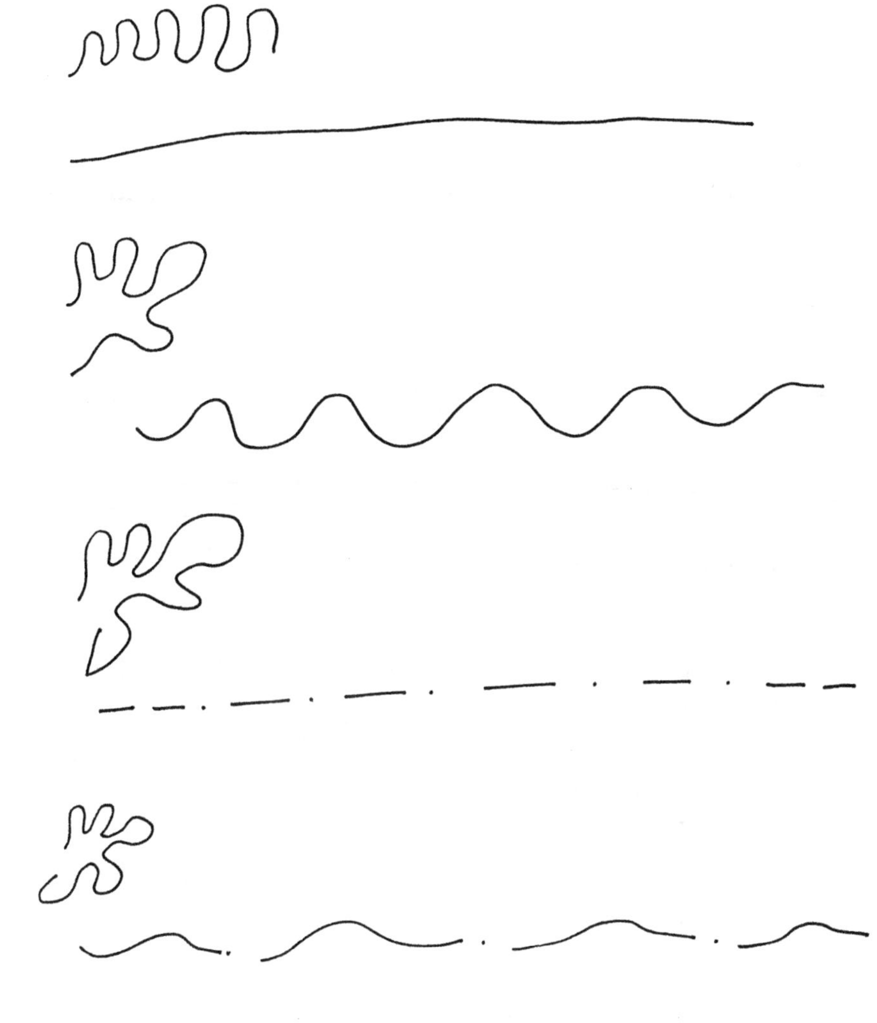

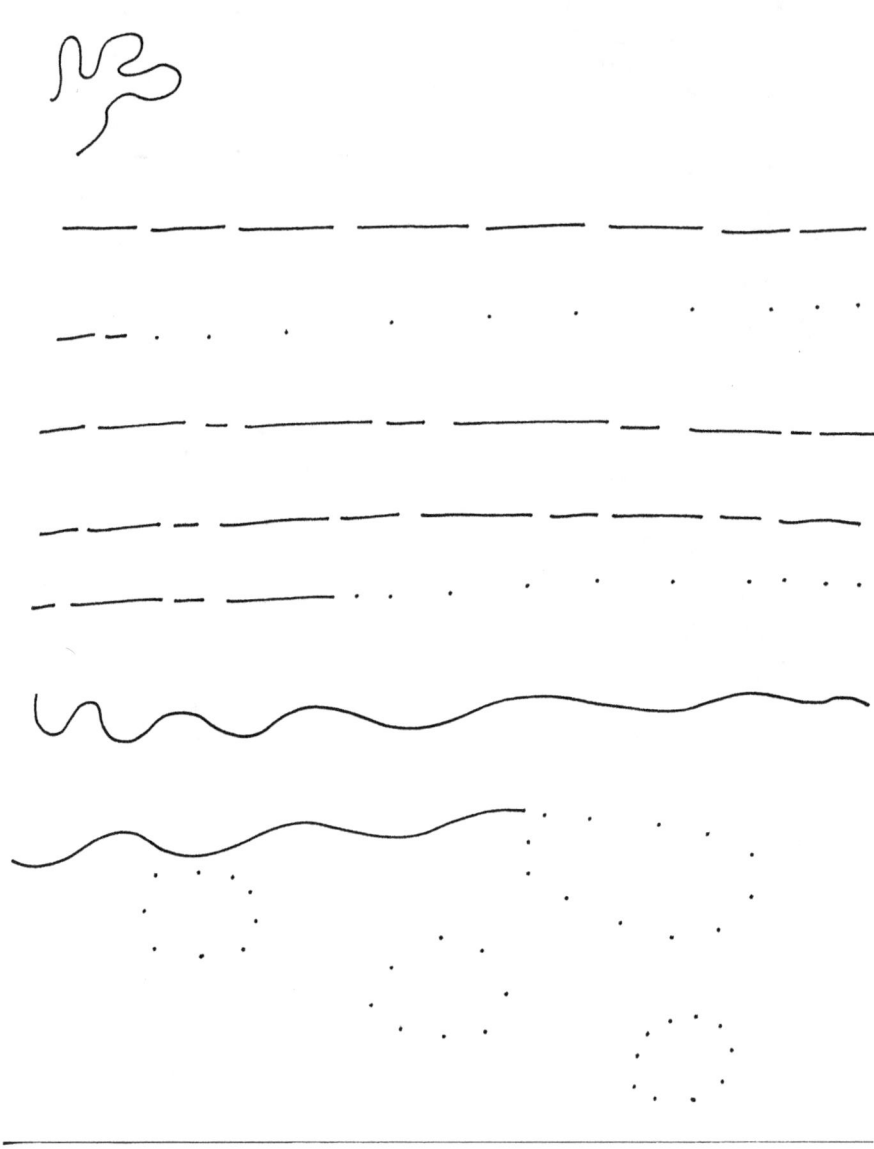

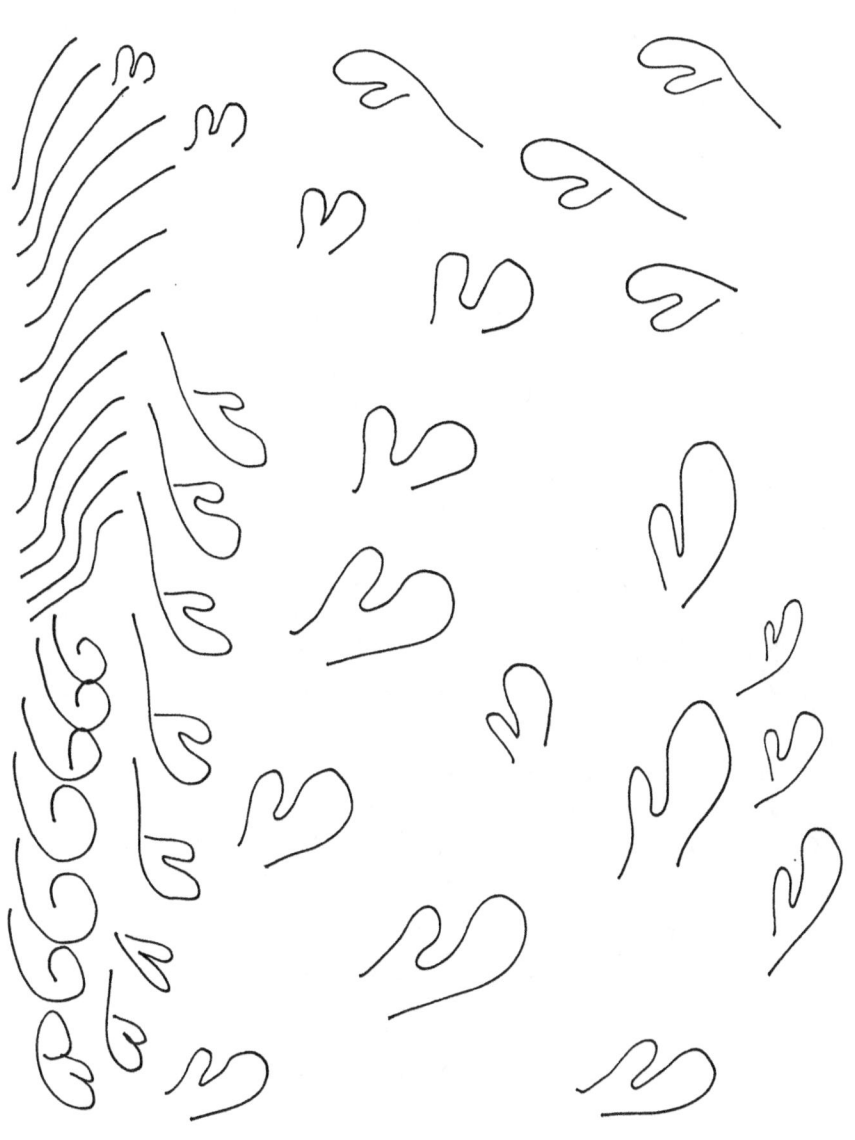

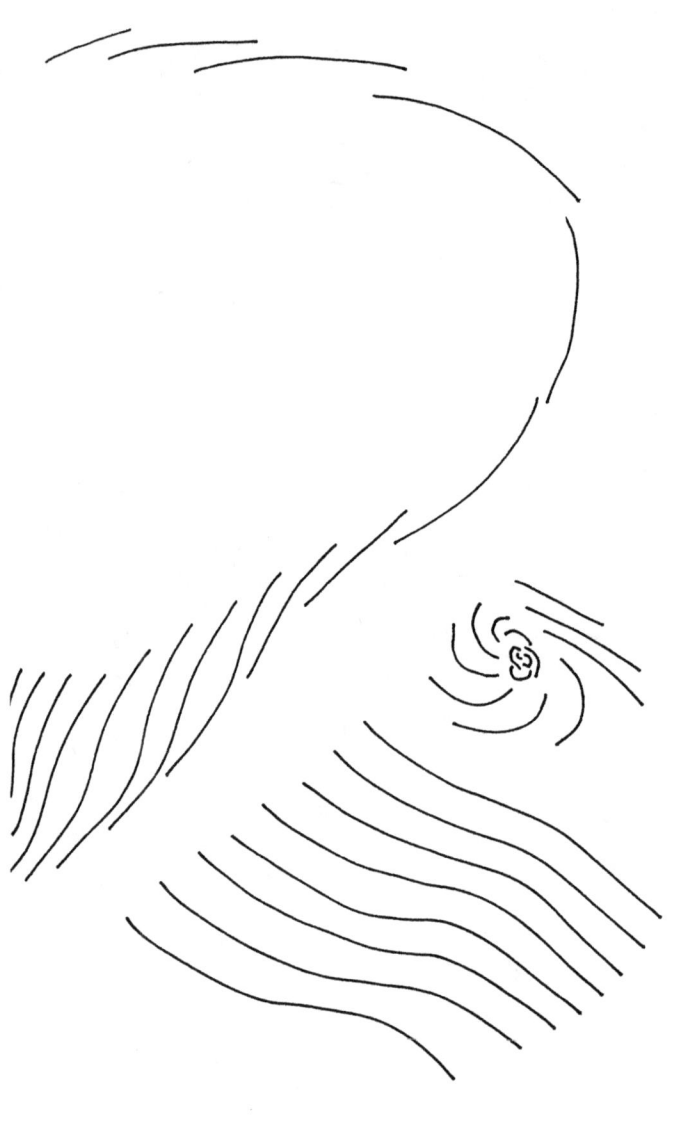

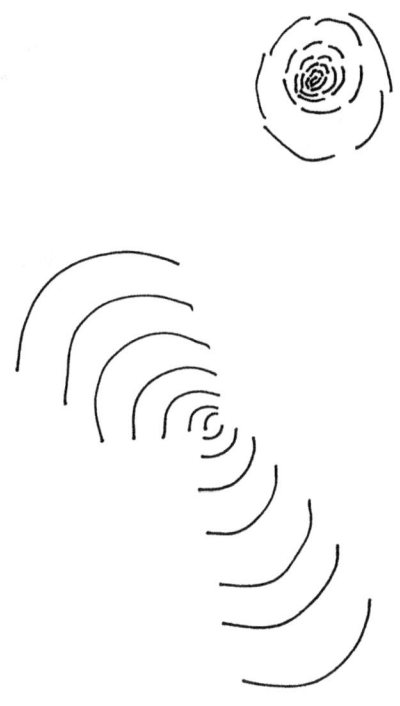

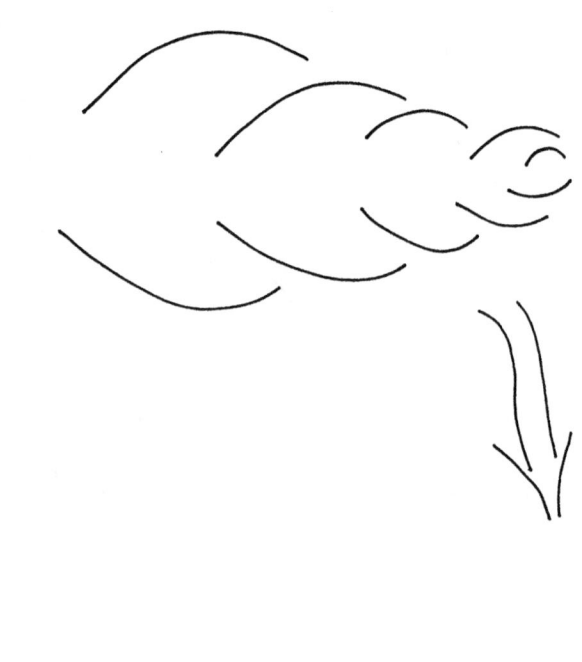

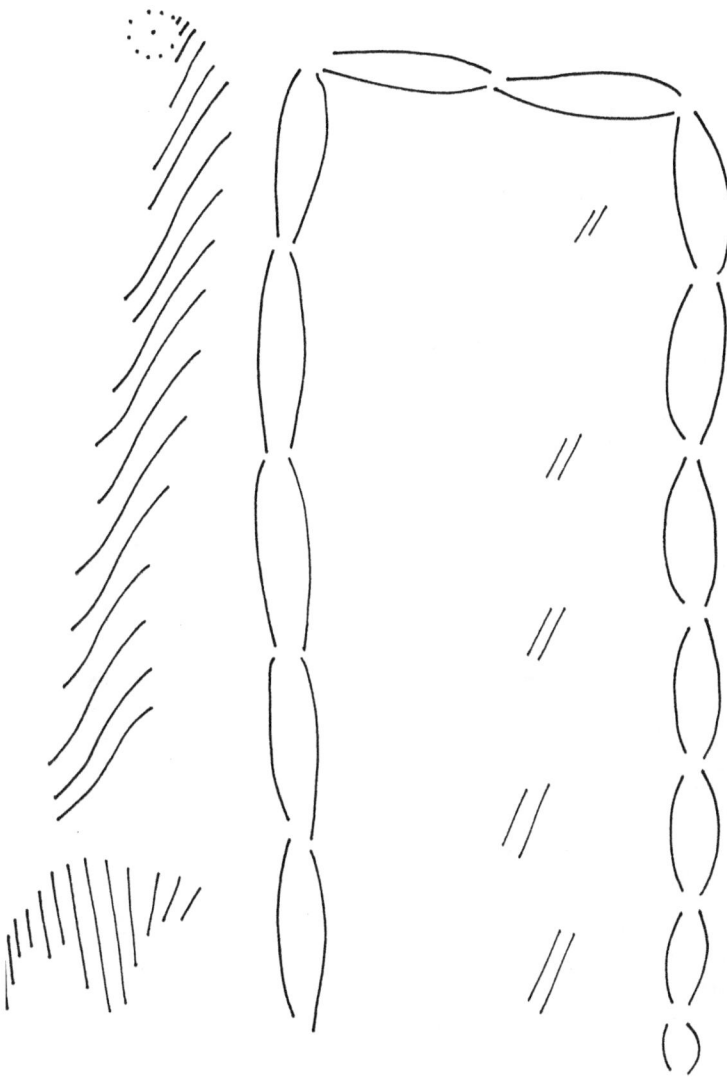

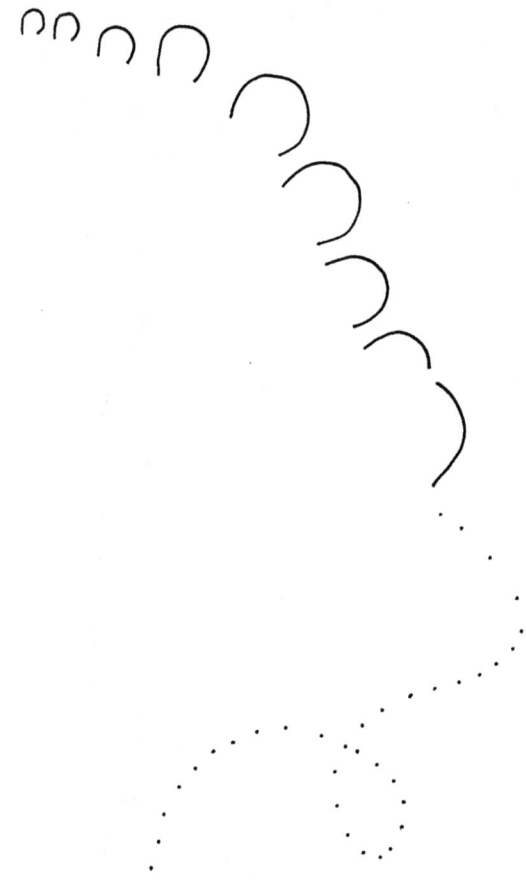

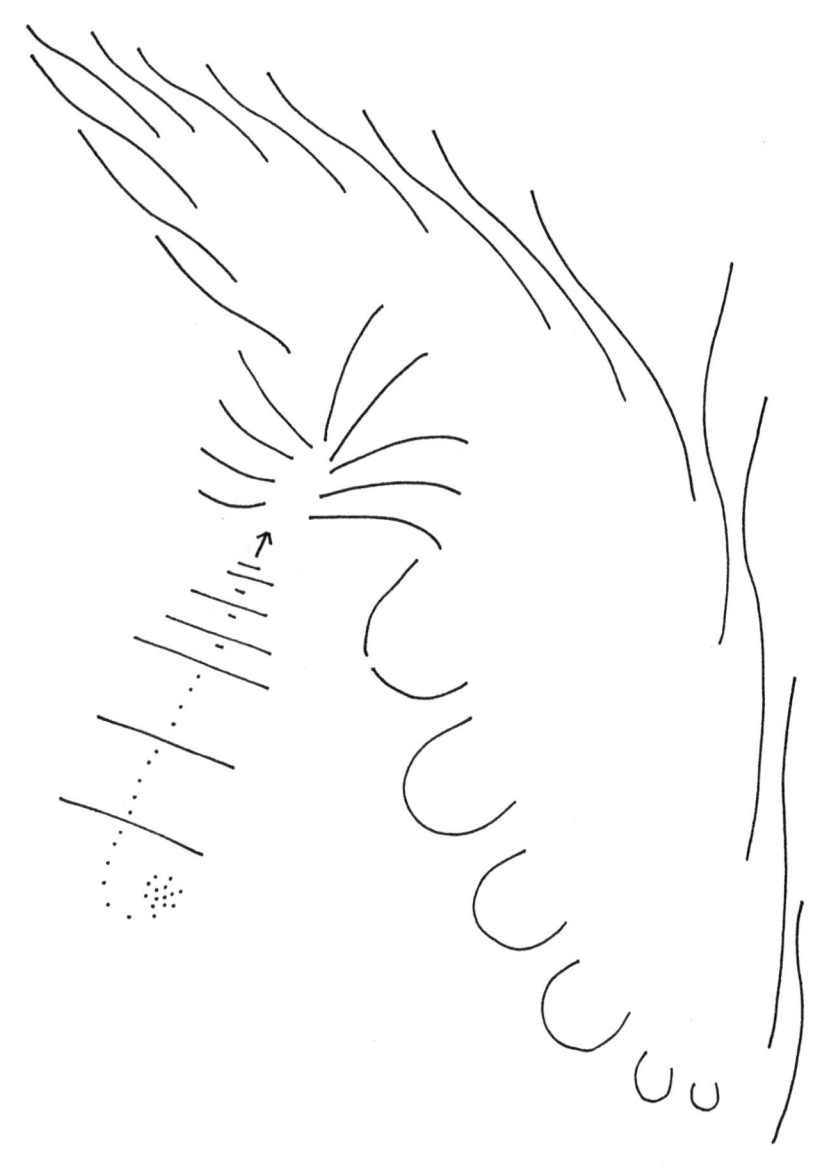

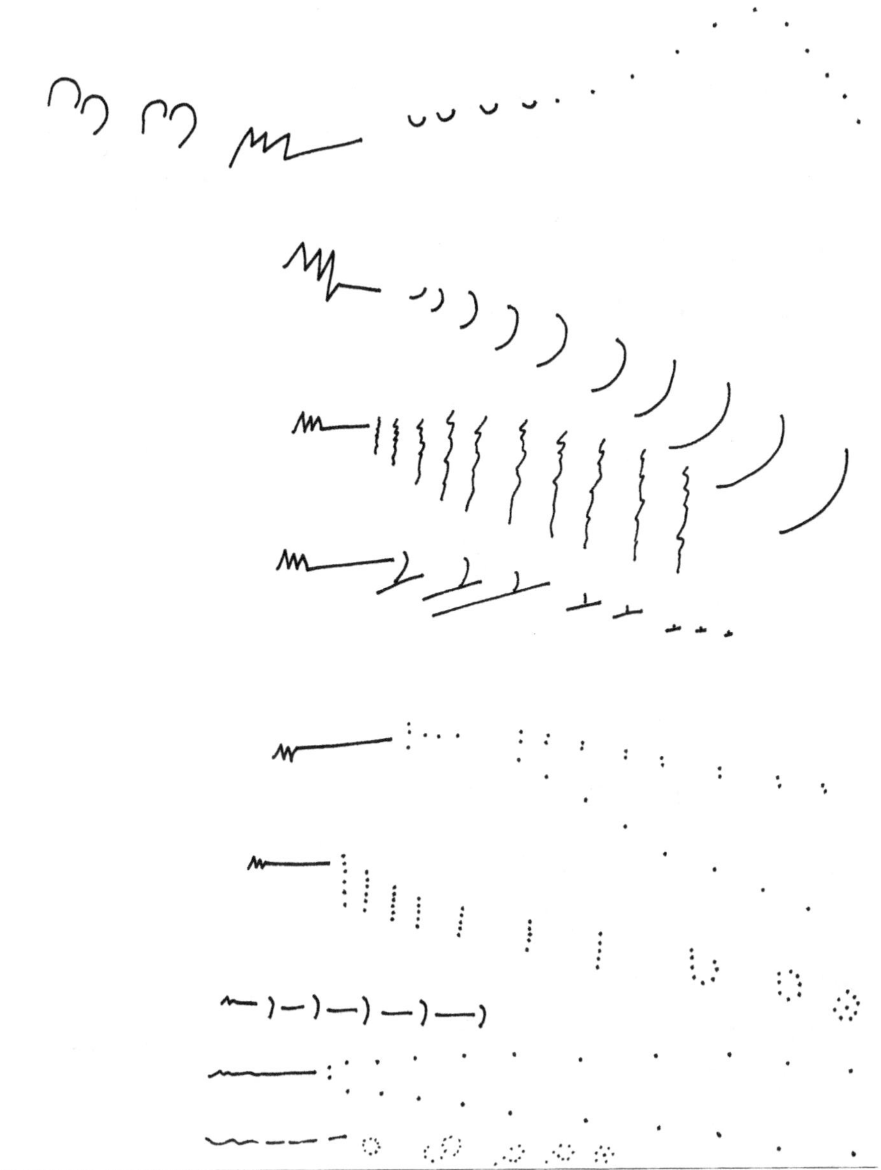

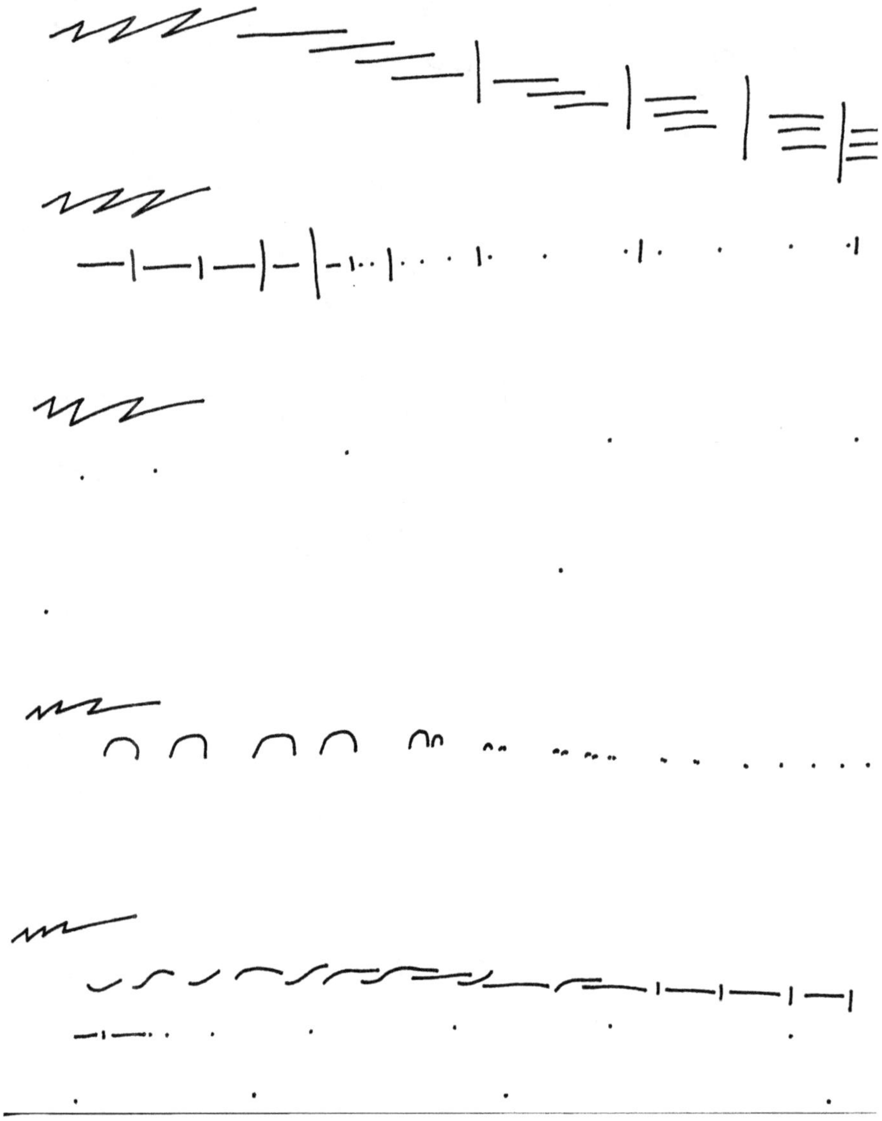

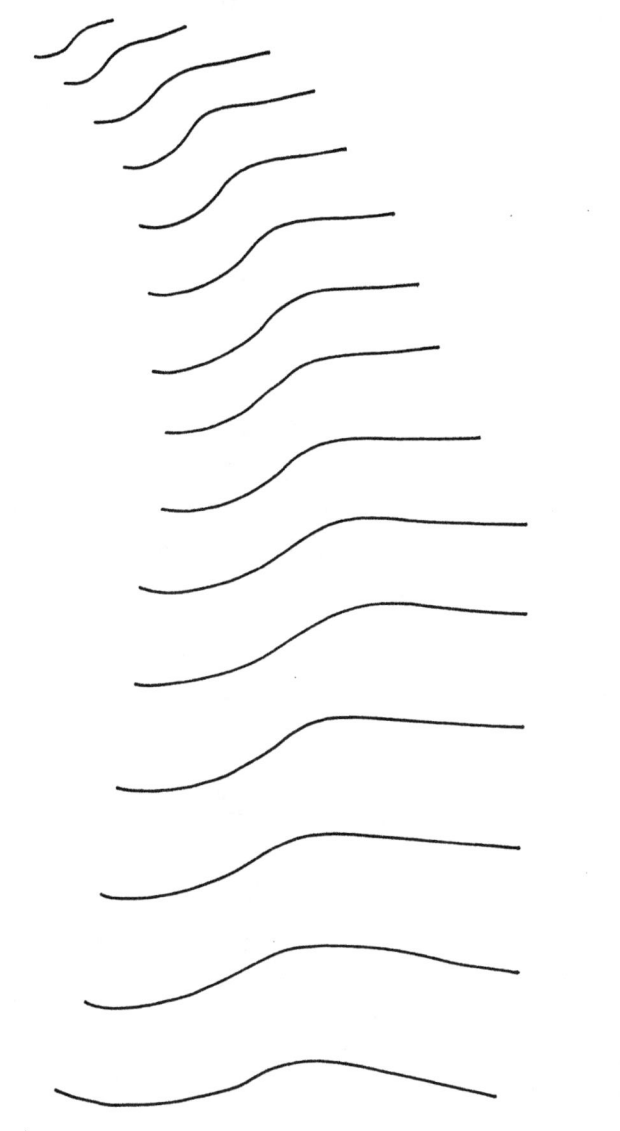

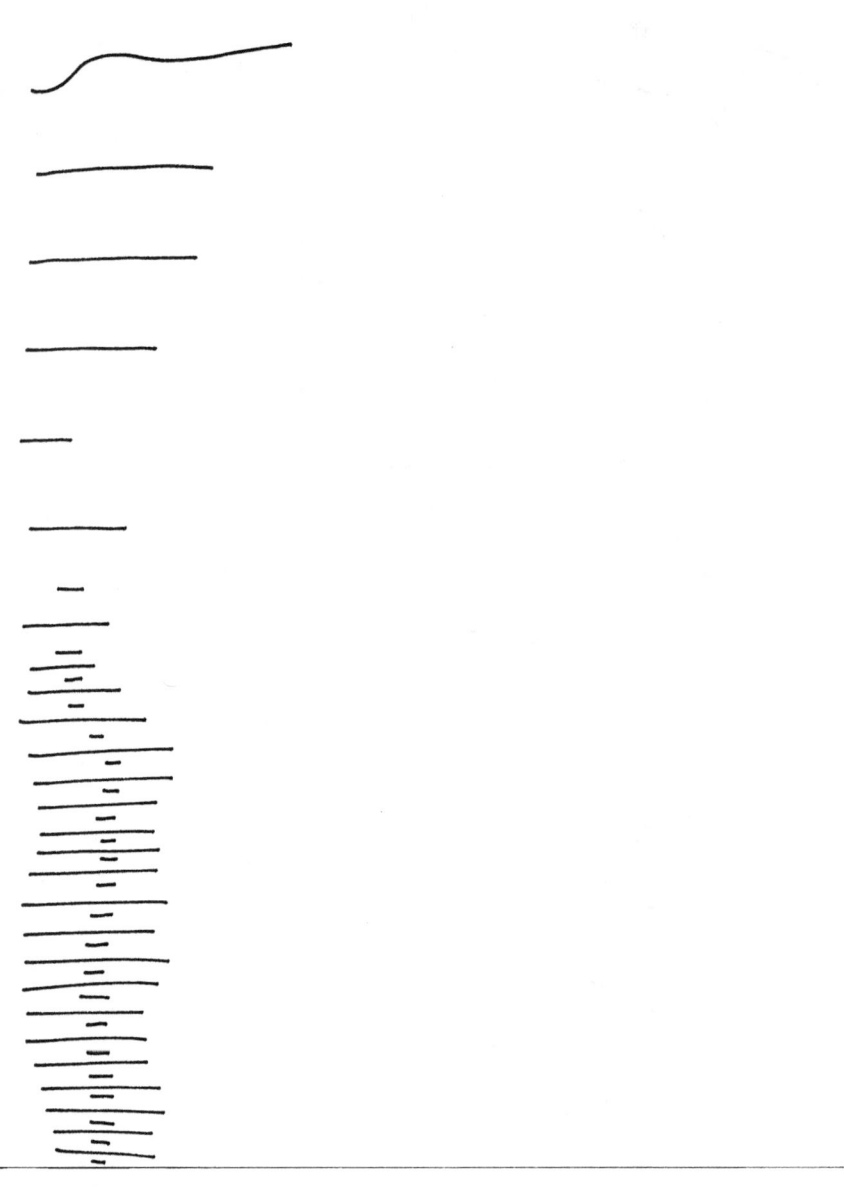

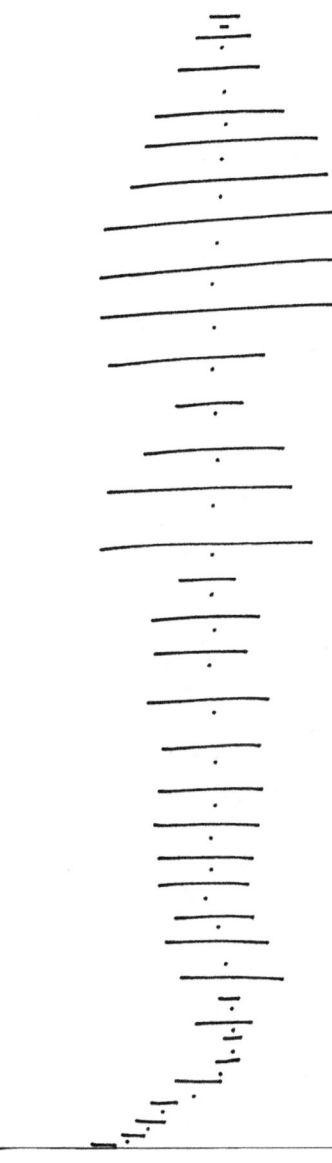

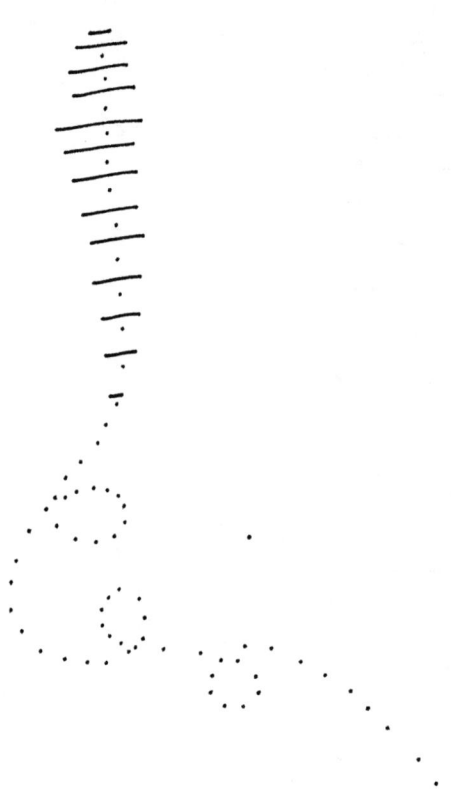

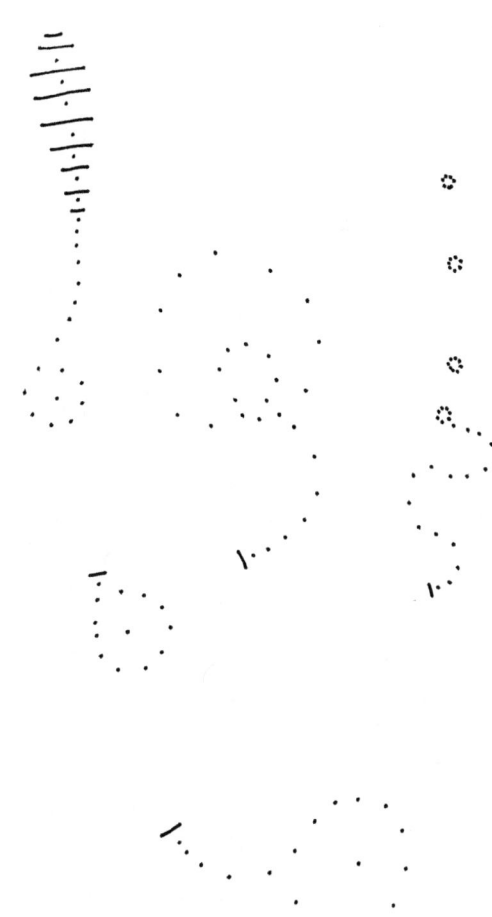

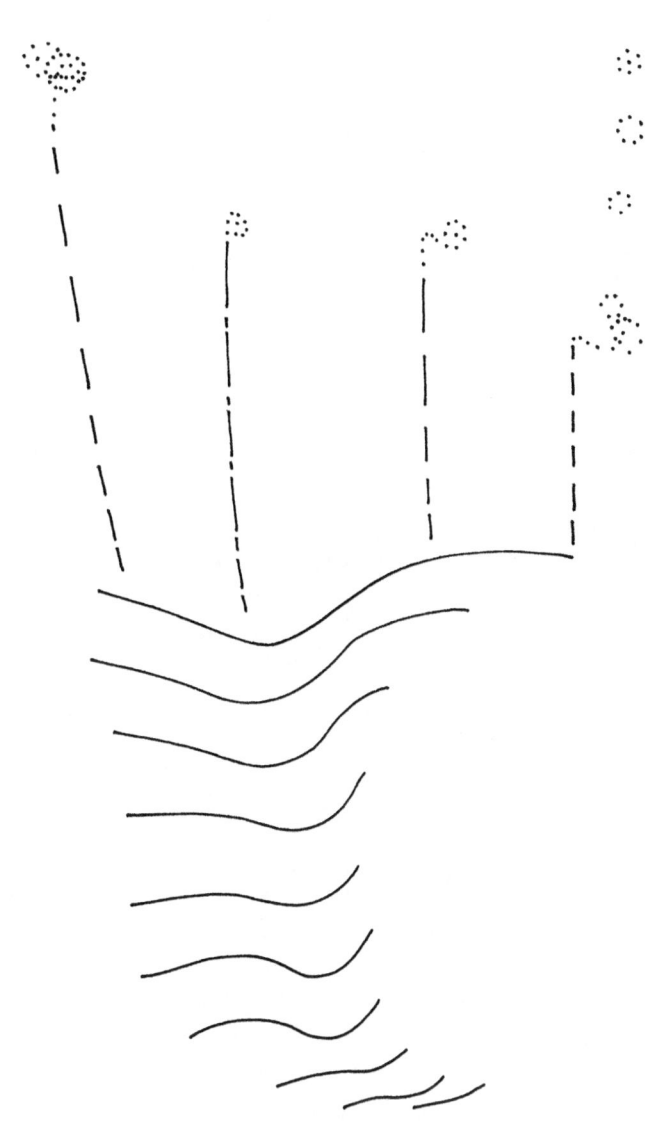

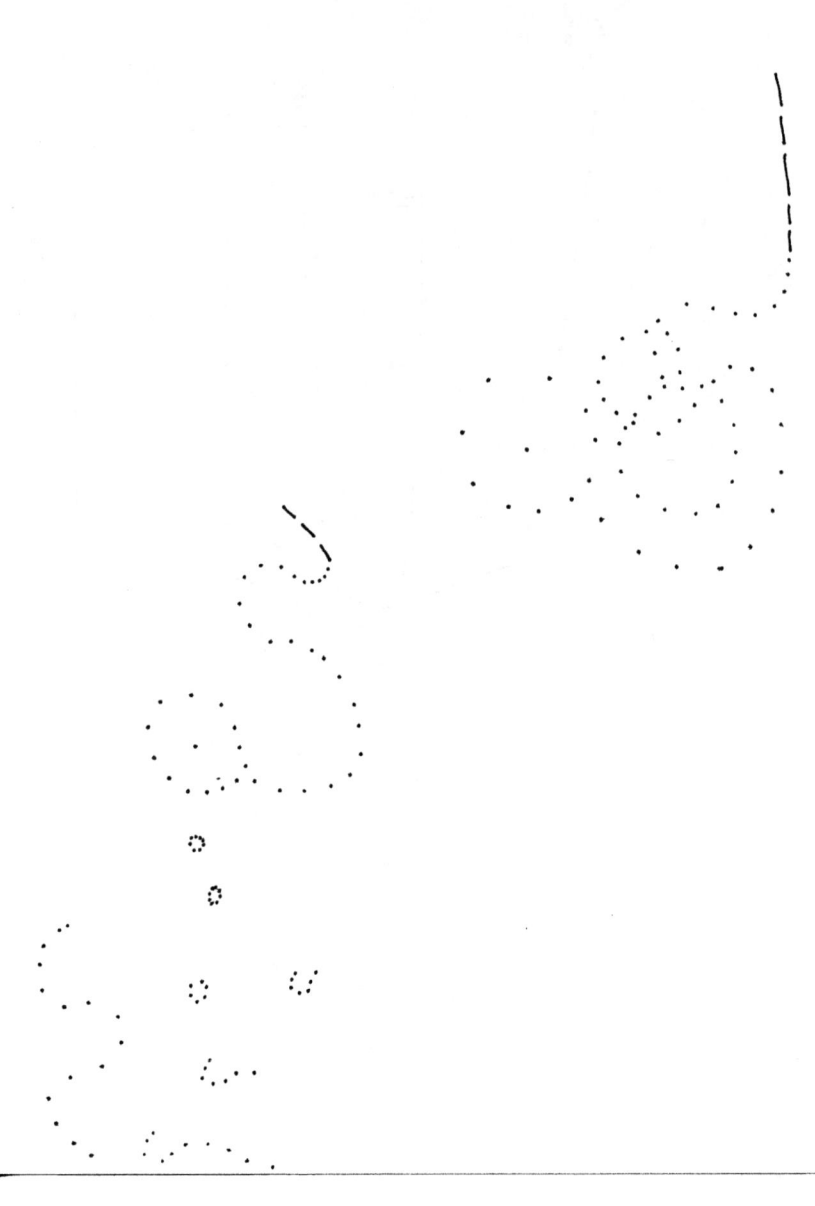

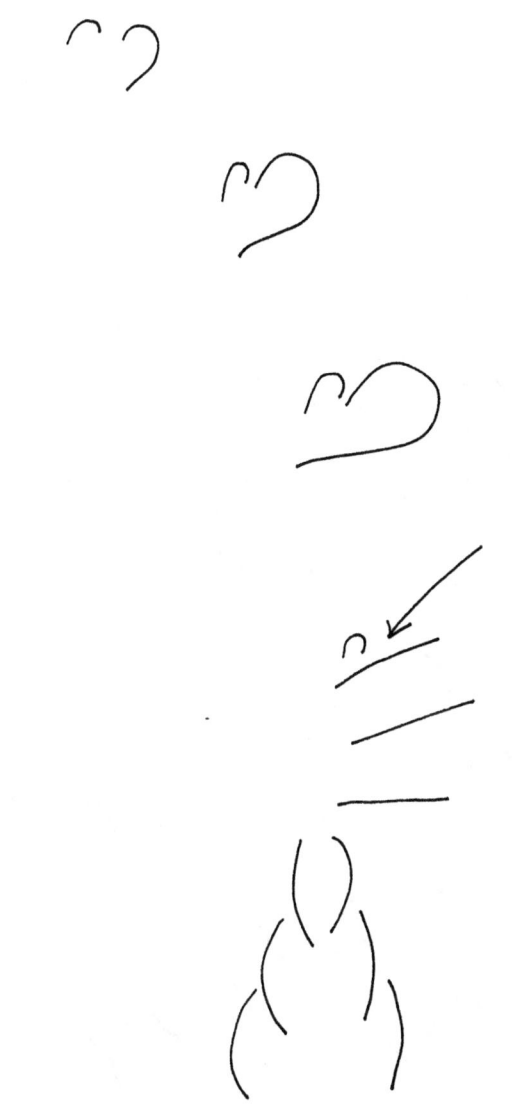

c   √

c

✓

c

✓

c

c

c

C

c

✓

c

✓

c

c

√

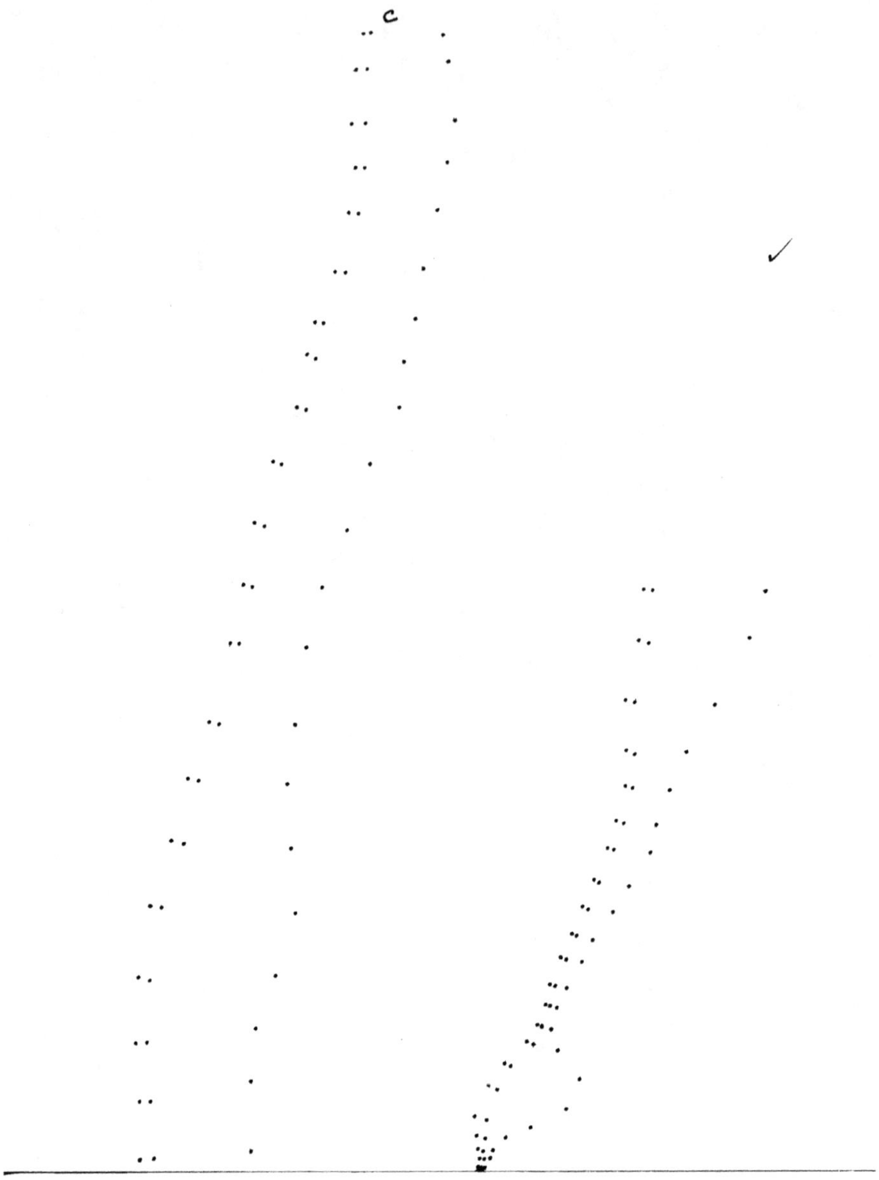
c

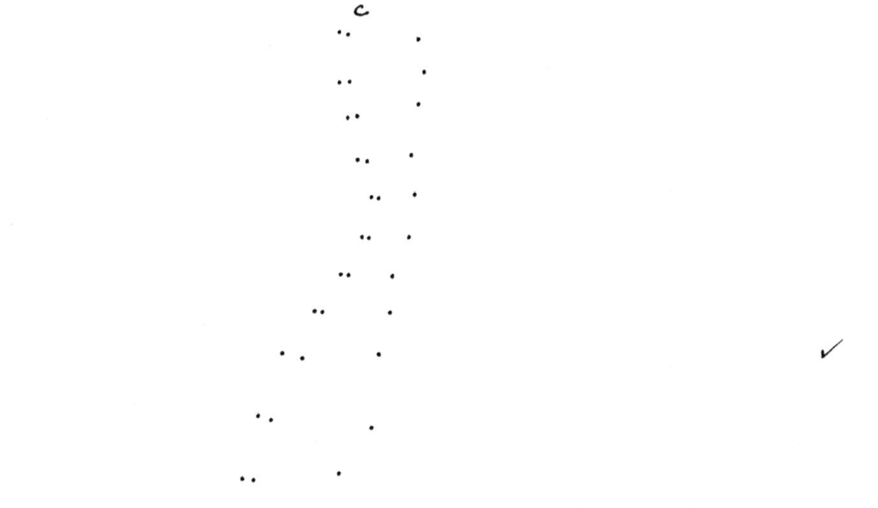
c

c

c

c

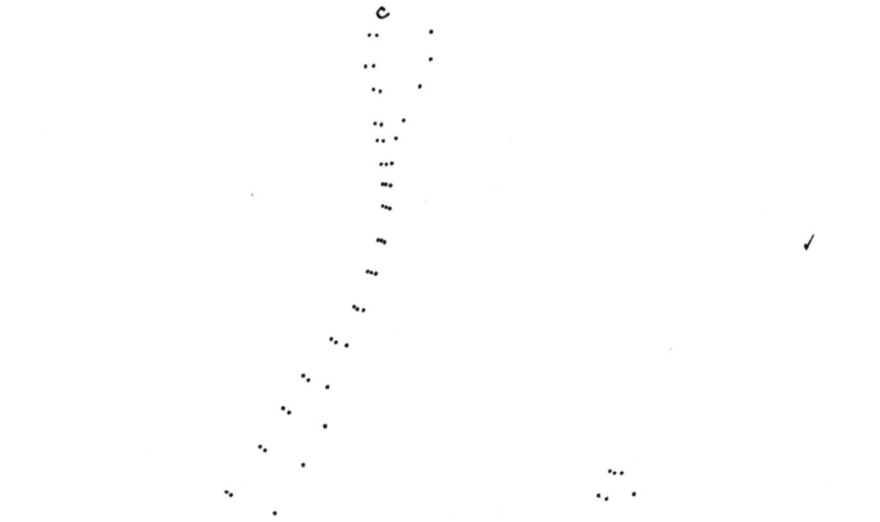
c

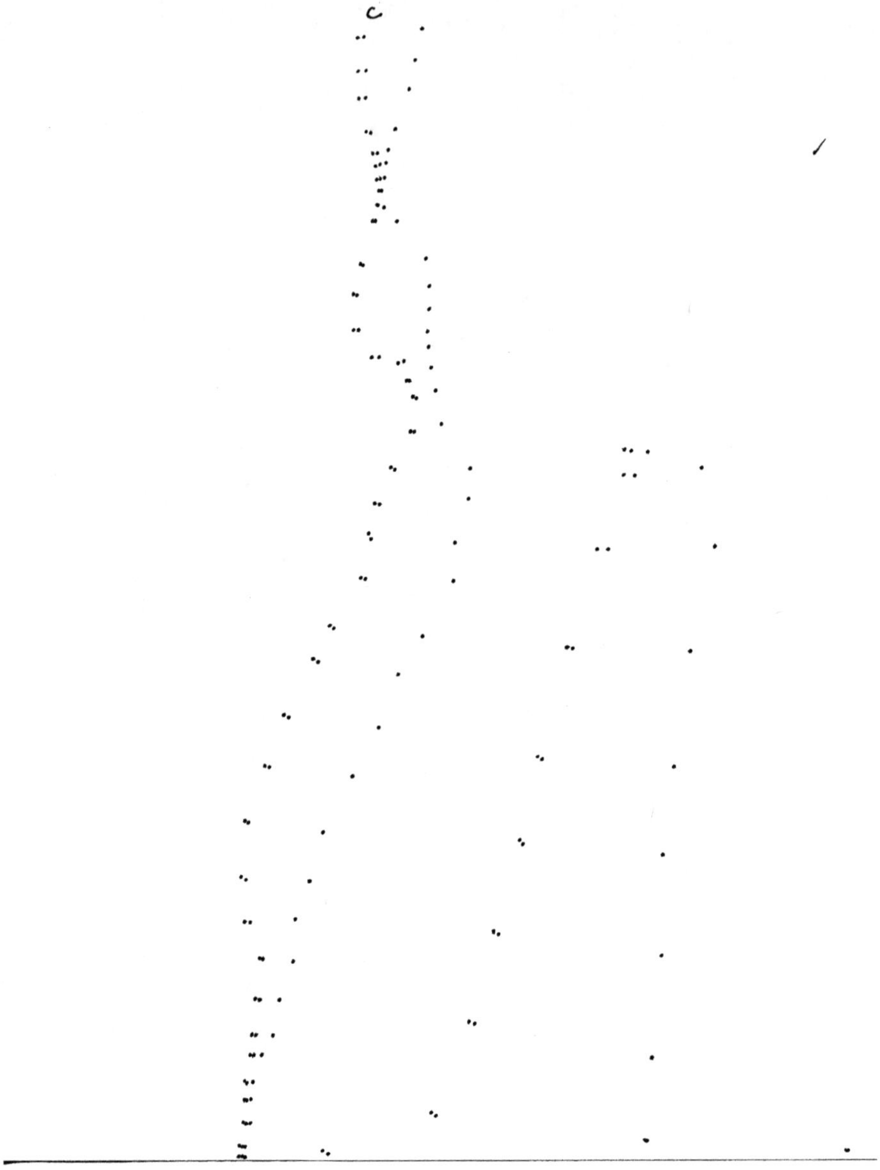

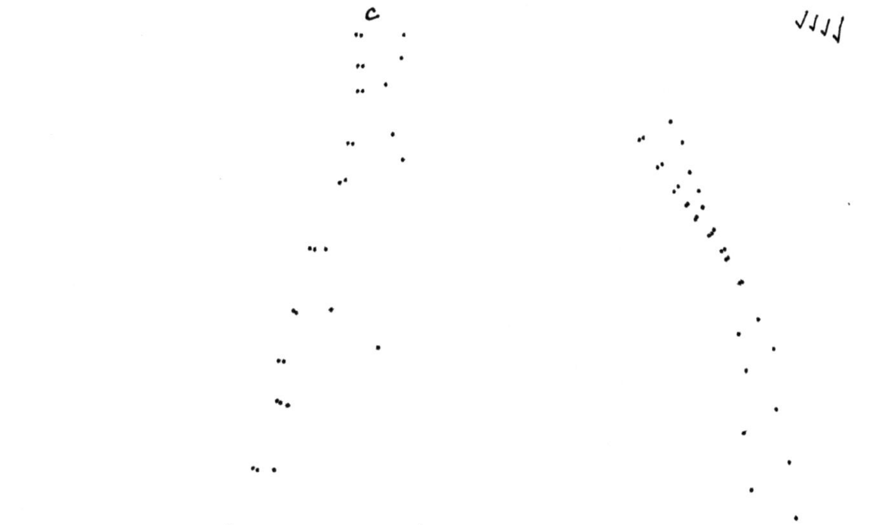

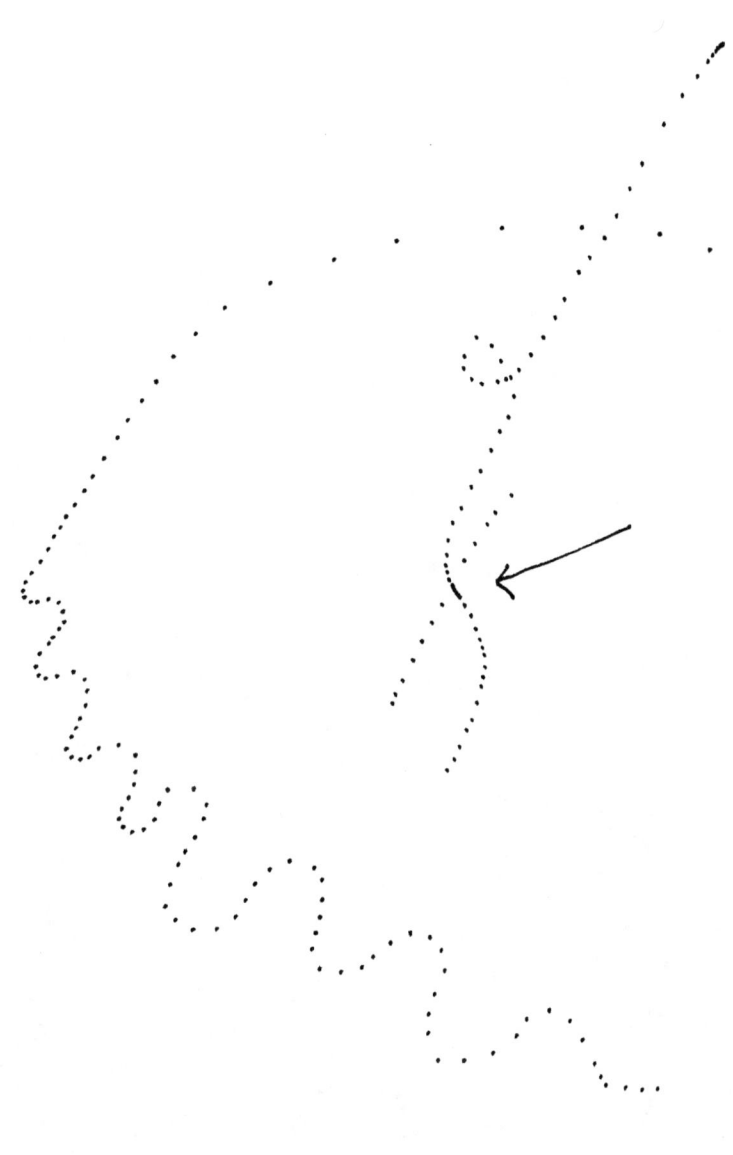

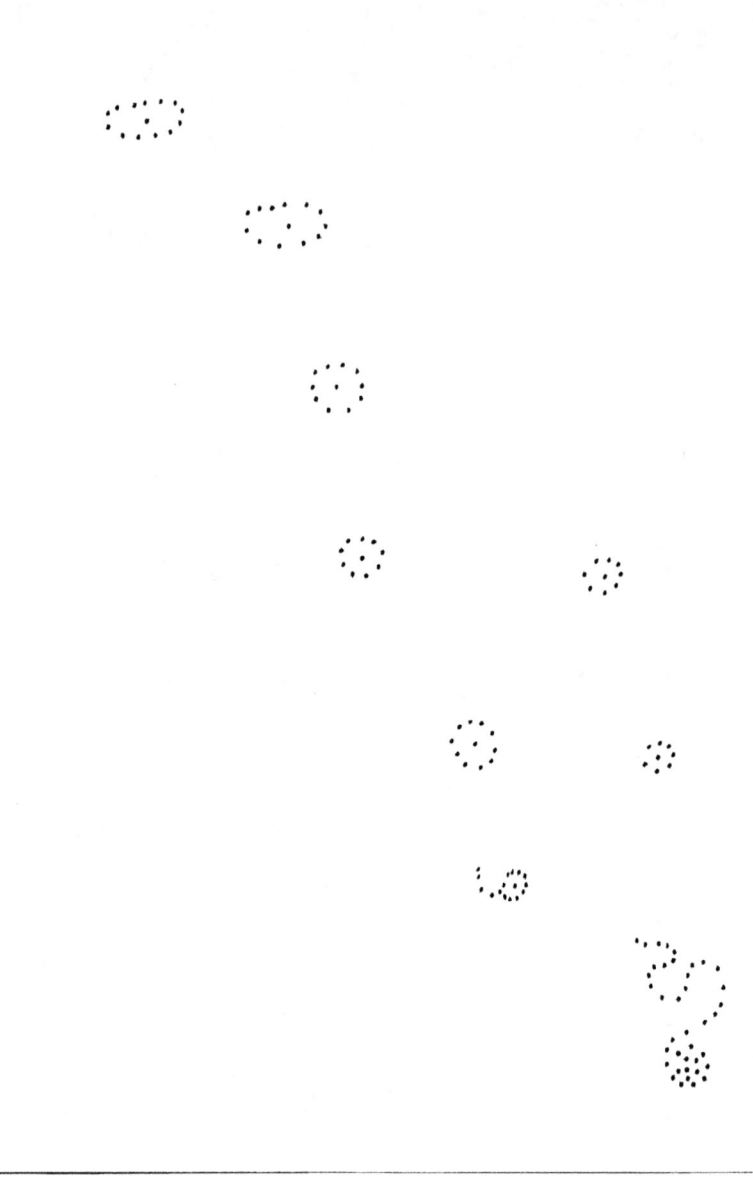

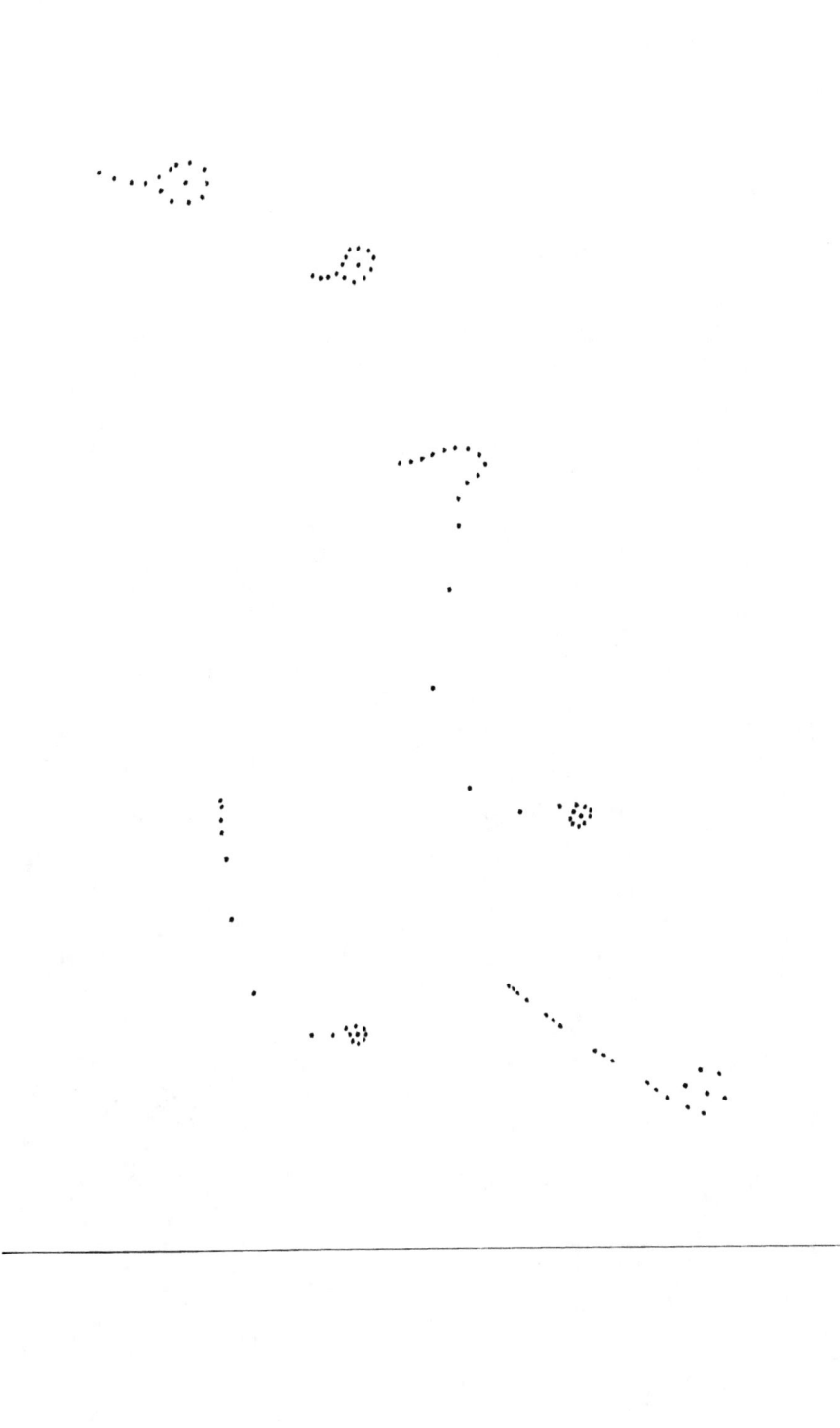

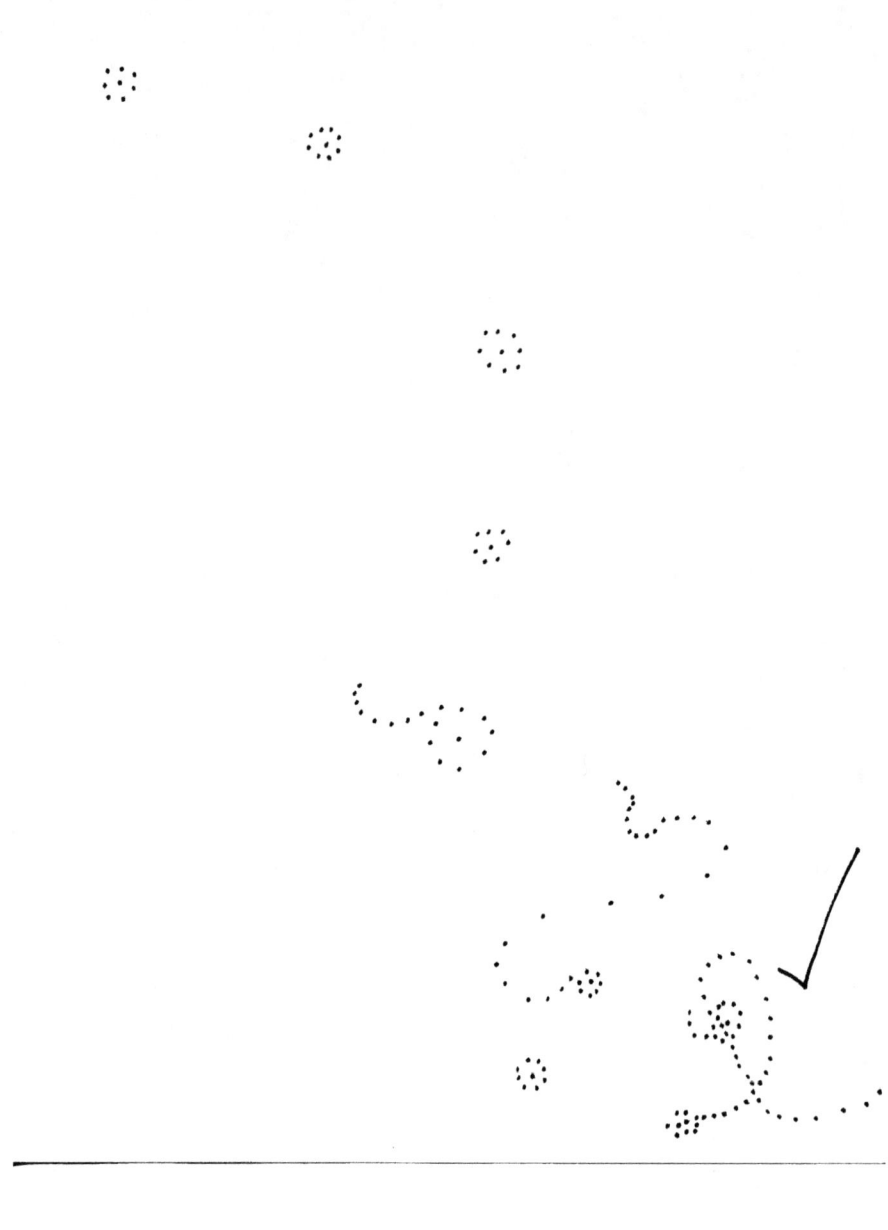

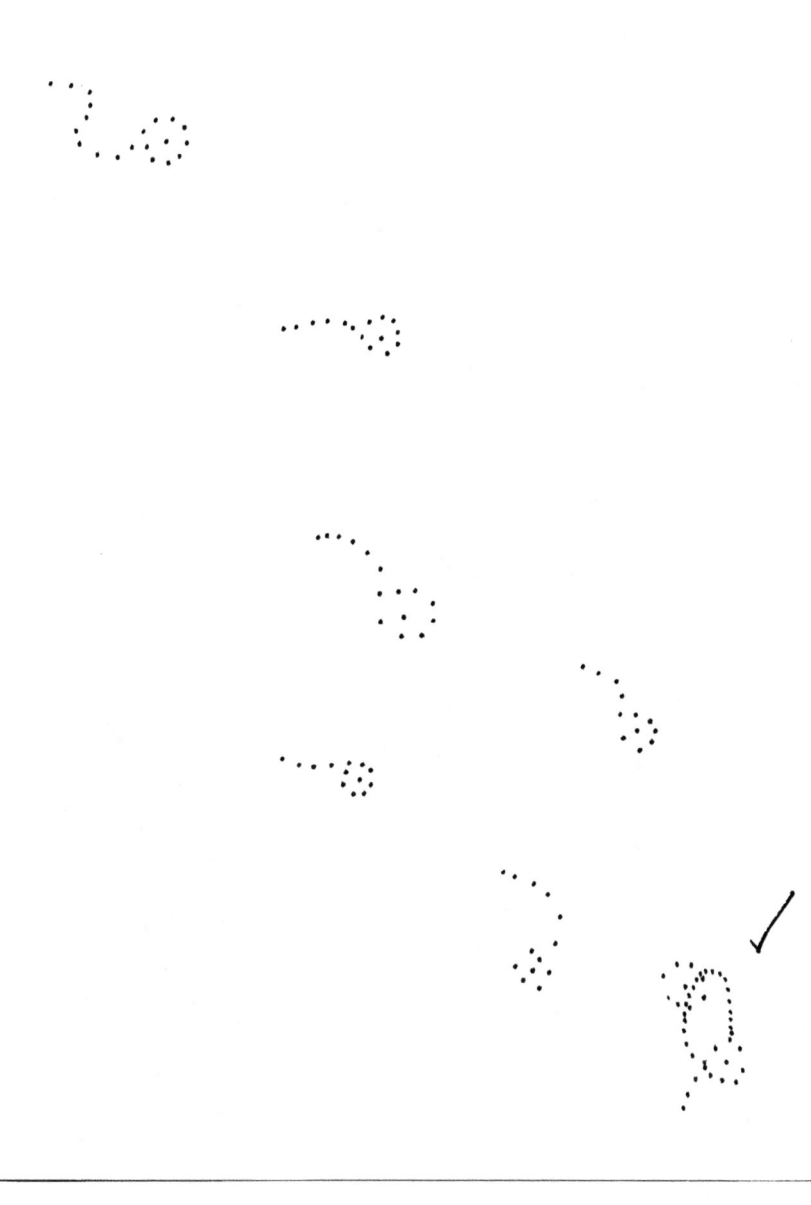

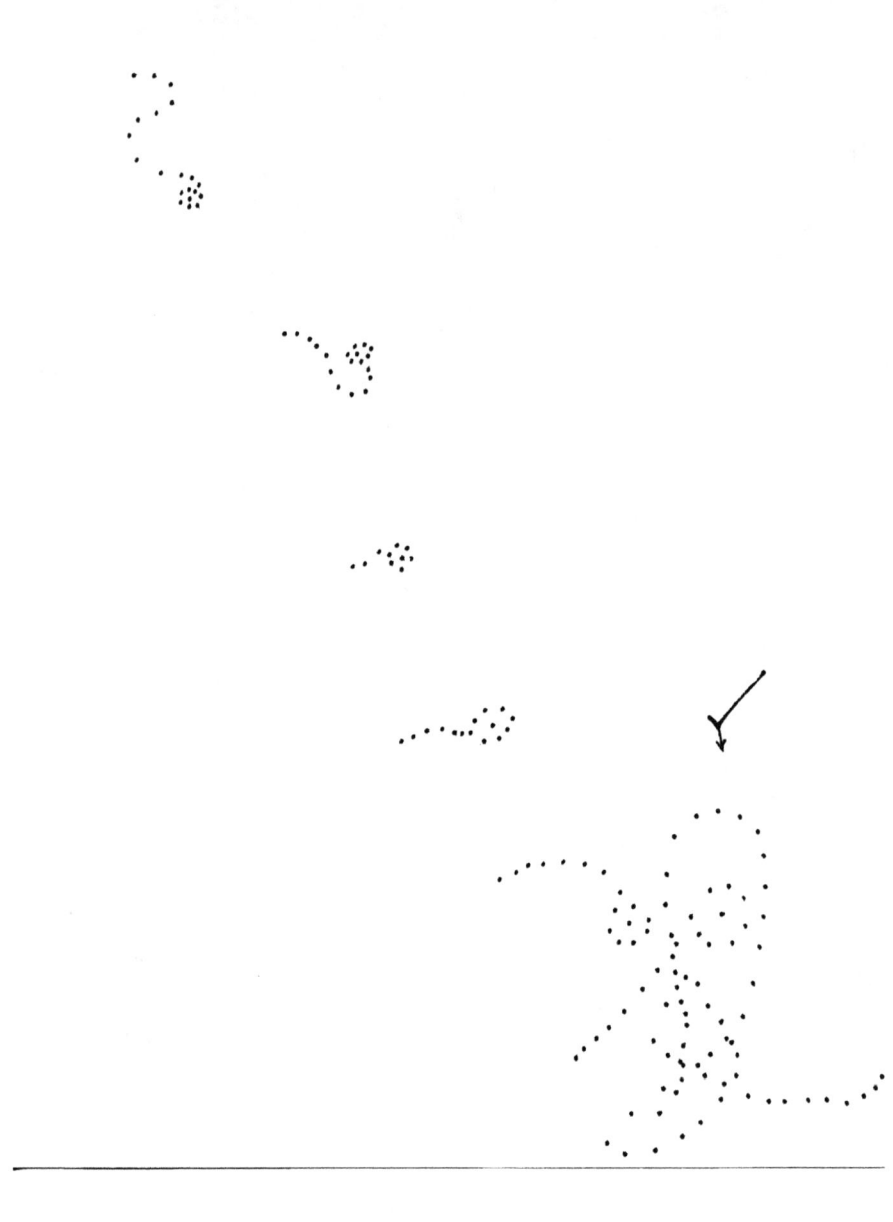

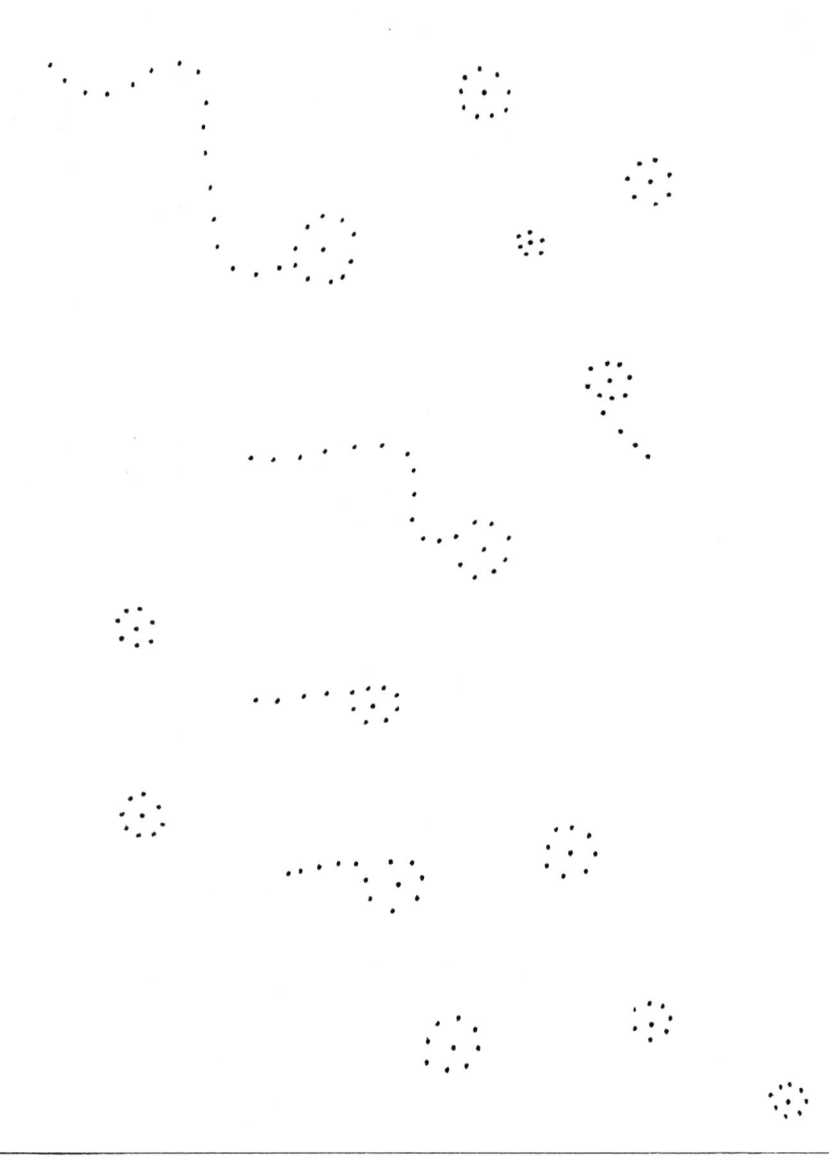

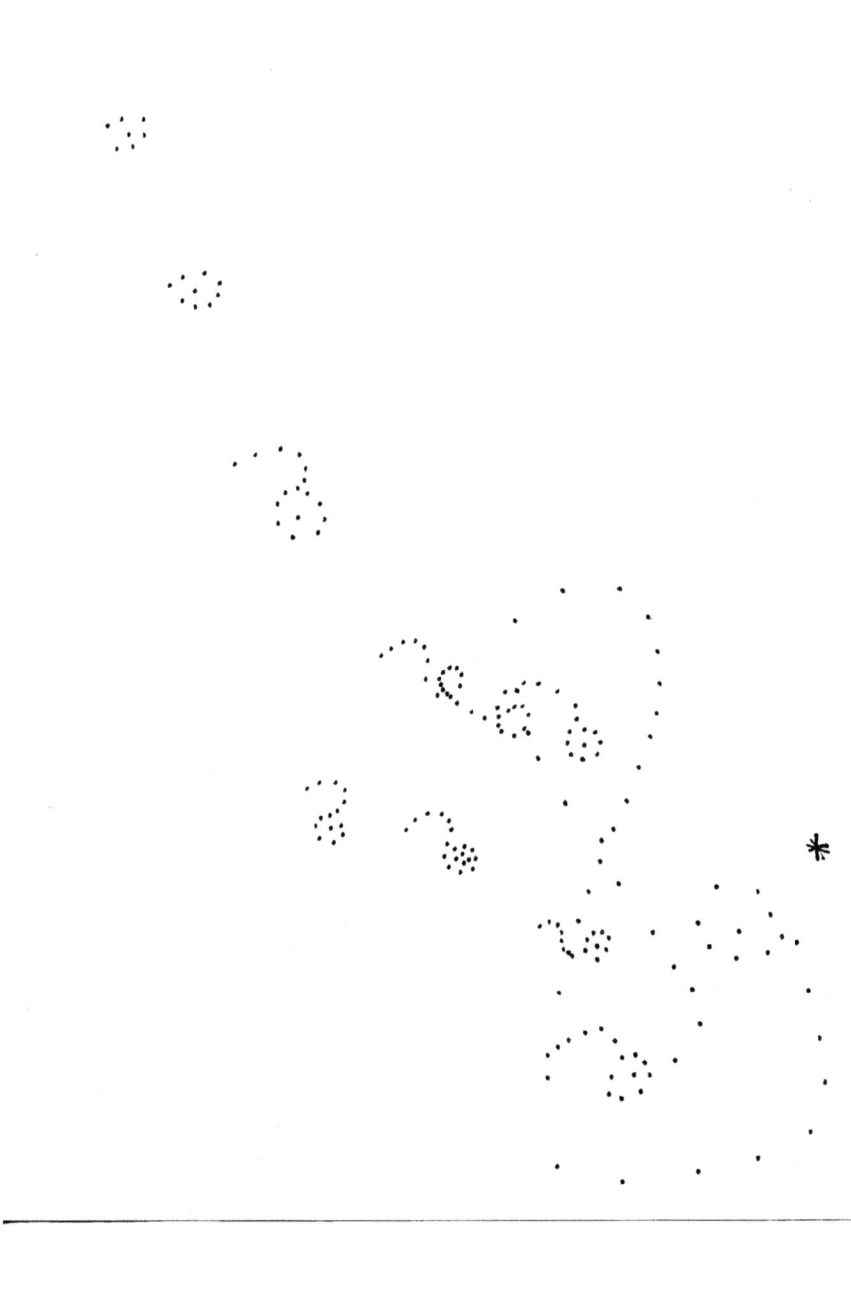

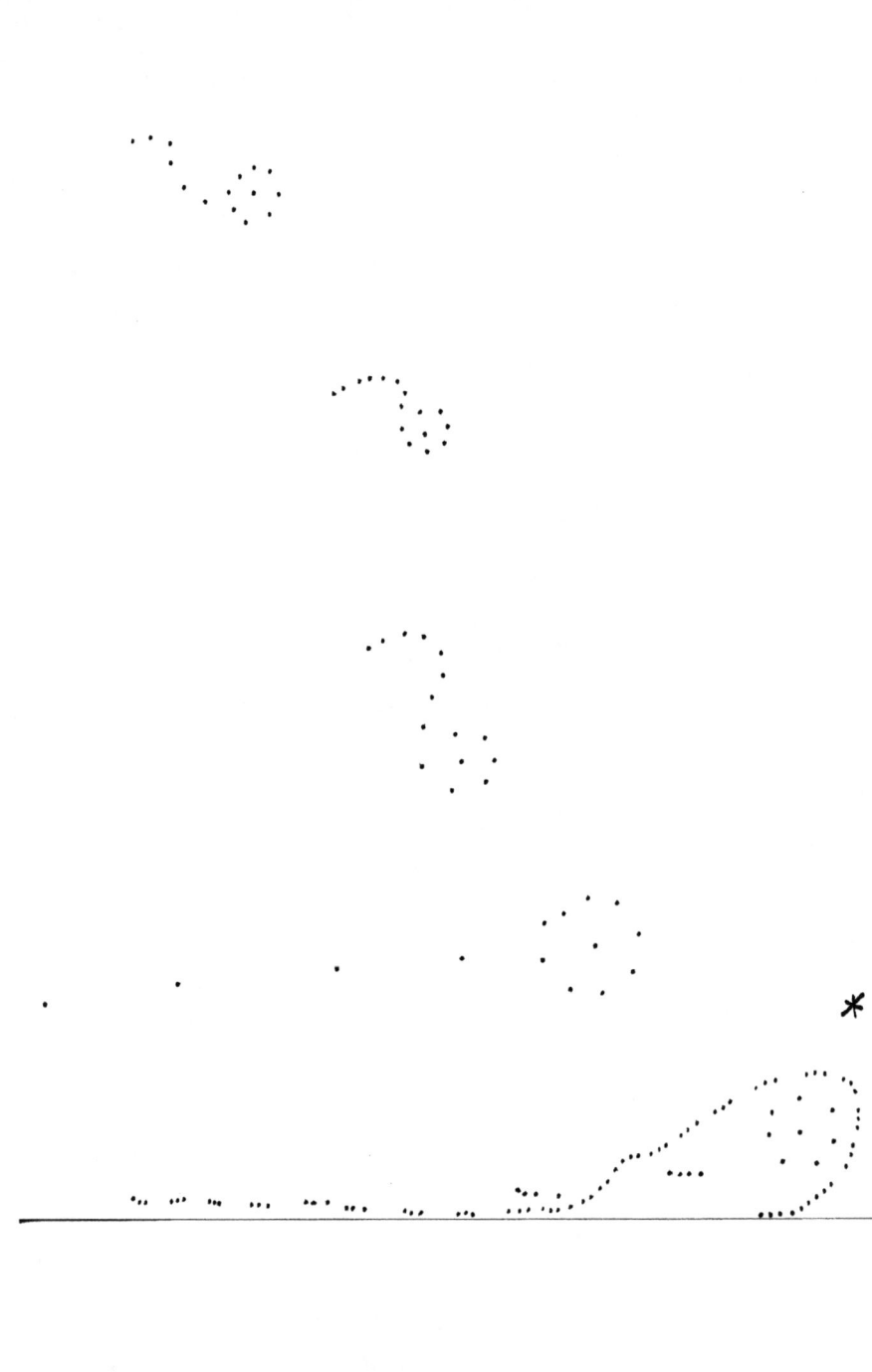